C000143490

50 TIPS
TO BUILD YOUR
SELF-ESTEEM

50 TIPS TO BUILD YOUR SELF-ESTEEM

Summersdale Publishers Ltd
46 West Street
Chichester
West Sussex
PO19 1RP
UK

www.summersdale.com

Printed and bound in the Czech Republic

ISBN: 978-1-84953-509-0

Substantial discounts on bulk quantities of Summersdale books are available to corporations, professional associations and other organisations. For details contact Nicky Douglas by telephone: +44 (0) 1243 756902, fax: +44 (0) 1243 786300 or email: nicky@summersdale.com.

50 TIPS
TO BUILD YOUR
SELF-ESTEEM

Anna Barnes

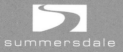

summersdale

Introduction

Self-esteem is a key component to a happy, successful life. Self-esteem is essentially how you feel about yourself in terms of your personal qualities and traits, your skills and abilities. Someone with high self-esteem will focus more on their positive traits and see themselves as a capable and talented individual, whereas someone with low self-esteem will likely feel generally unworthy.

This book provides easy-to-follow tips to help boost your self-esteem and get you feeling good about yourself. If, however, you feel your self-esteem is so low it is strongly affecting your day-to-day life, it is advised that you seek advice from your doctor.

SECTION ONE:

UNDERSTANDING SELF-ESTEEM

To be able to improve a situation, you must first understand it. Knowing what triggers feelings of low self-esteem, and what makes you feel good about yourself and your abilities, is the best place to start from to act upon building your self-esteem.

Talk to friends and family

Sometimes it can be hard to know exactly what is causing our self-esteem to be low and in these cases, one of the best things you can do is speak to a good friend or a family member. If you can vocalise your concerns it may help you to understand where it is coming from, and if the person you choose to confide in knows you well, they may be able to offer you some insight that perhaps you have not been able to identify. Finally, talking is a positive and cathartic action, and simply airing your concerns can make you feel calmer and more ready for coming challenges. Added to that, your friends and family tend to think well of you, and hearing positive remarks from them can be a real boost to your self-confidence.

2

See your self-esteem grow

When you start your journey towards stronger self-esteem, it can be hard to see what the end result will be. It is easy to be concerned about the 'what ifs' of a situation, and this is where visualisation can help. Sitting in a comfortable chair, in a relaxed position, close your eyes and begin to focus on your breathing. There is no need to breathe more slowly or deeply, just pay attention to your natural breathing patterns. Next, start to build a picture in your head of how you would look and act with high self-esteem. Where are you? Who is with you? Notice the details and enjoy the feeling of confidence and happiness. While you are working on building your self-esteem, take this image with you and see it as something to look forward to.

3

Write down your worries

Once you have researched self-esteem, and have some idea of the issues and symptoms you are looking out for, it's time to work out what your personal triggers are, and when your self-esteem is at its highest or lowest points. Choose a notebook that reflects your tastes; anything from a simple notepad to an illustrated diary. Having a book which you like the look and feel of will make you more likely to use it. Keep it where you are most likely to use it – by the bed, in the kitchen – wherever you think you will pick it up and write in it. The act of writing down how you feel at any given time will not only help you keep track of what may cause a bout of low self-esteem, it is also cathartic. Furthermore, the diary gives you something to look back at on days when you feel low, which shows that things can be better.

SECTION TWO:

EAT HEALTHILY, FEEL GREAT

Feeding your body the right foods in the right quantities, and ensuring you include mood-boosting nutrients, is a great way to lift your self-esteem by making you feel healthier on the inside, and helping you look your best on the outside. Use these simple tips to boost your nutrition and your mood.

4

Getting the balance right

Whilst certain foods are said to help with specific things, such as being good for the heart or digestion, the most important thing to start with is a balanced, healthy diet which incorporates all the major food groups. Once you have ensured that you are getting enough protein, fibre, fat, and plenty of vitamin-rich fruits and vegetables, you have a great starting point for healthy eating, which will make you feel fantastic inside and out. If you are unsure of the foods that are best for optimum health, a web search will provide you with comprehensive lists of which foods are rich in which nutrients, allowing you to plan healthier meals.

5

Try a low GI for steady energy

You may have heard about the health benefits of a low-GI diet – more steady energy levels, less bloating, no sugar cravings – all of which can be beneficial for your self-esteem. GI stands for Glycaemic Index; the ranking of carbohydrate-containing foods based on their overall effect on blood glucose levels. When we eat foods with a high GI, such as white bread, pastries and sweets, our blood sugar spikes and then drops rapidly, leaving us tired, irritable and hungry. Eating low-GI foods – such as beans, rye breads and most fruit and veg – helps to ensure your body is fuelled throughout the day and night, leaving you feeling more balanced.

6

Pep up with protein

As well as being essential for building muscle, protein is important for managing hunger levels and for improving mood. Proteins are made up of amino acids; the essential building blocks from which our body produces almost everything. In particular, the amino acids tryptophan and phenylalanine are great for the mood, as they are used in the production of the neurotransmitters serotonin, dopamine and adrenaline. These three hormones help you to feel happier and more motivated naturally.

7

Be fat friendly

When trying to eat healthily, it can be easy to see fat as the enemy. Many 'healthy' products are marketed as low fat or fat-free, and we are led to believe that eating fat makes you fat. This is, however, not entirely true. Fats are an important part of your diet. They are key in neurotransmitter production due to the amino acids they contain, and unsaturated fats are important for healthy skin and hair. As long as you get the balance right and are eating enough monounsaturated and polyunsaturated fats, such as those found in olive oil and seeds, and you are reducing the amount of saturated fat you consume, for example the fats in butter, cheese and red meat, you can begin to benefit physically, and the positive changes in your appearance and general health can give you a boost emotionally.

Be naturally sweet

Low self-esteem can lead us to make poor food choices as we try to find comfort from food; sweet foods such as cake and chocolate offer the short-term surge of energy you may crave. Snacking on sugar-rich foods can have a very negative effect on the body both physically and emotionally; the inevitable weight gain can make you feel unhappy with your body, and has the potential to make you feel you have 'given in' to certain foods. This can be a cause of stress, which in turn can lead us to reach for sugary foods again, forming a vicious cycle.

Our modern lifestyles, however, mean that our stress is more likely to be because of bills we have to pay, or meetings we have to arrange, and reaching for the sugar is unhelpful because we do not really need the energy boost. Try chewing sugar-free gum, particularly if it is sweetened with natural xylitol, to give your body the taste of something sweet it is craving, without putting excess sugar that you will not use into your body.

9

Be ACE

Feeling low, especially long term, can cause higher stress levels and therefore raise levels of stress hormones in your system, which can have a negative effect on your health either by lowering your immune system, making you more prone to coughs, colds and other infections, or by over-stimulating it and provoking autoimmune illnesses and inflammation. A simple way to combat these symptoms is to eat plenty of foods rich in the antioxidant vitamins A, C and E. These antioxidants help normalise the body and reduce inflammation, whilst boosting immunity.

Vitamin A is found in the form of retinol in products such as fatty fish, liver and egg yolks. Too much retinol can be bad for health though, so balance this with beta-carotene, found in mainly yellow and orange fruits and vegetables such as carrots, butternut squash and apricots. Vitamin C is found in good amounts in citrus fruits, broccoli, berries and tomatoes, and vitamin E is found in, amongst others, cooked spinach, nuts, seeds, avocadoes, olive oil and wheatgerm. Adding some of these foods to your diet could make you feel healthier and happier.

10

Get a boost with B vitamins

The B vitamin group is particularly important for maintaining a balanced mood. Amongst their other functions, B vitamins are involved in the body's control of tryptophan, a building block for serotonin. Vitamin B6 is essential in the production of GABA (gamma-aminobutyric acid), which helps boost mood in a similar way to serotonin. A lack of these essential neurotransmitters can lead to low mood, which in turn can lead to very serious psychological problems. The main vitamins to pay attention to are B1, B3, B5, B6, B9 and B12, all of which can be found in a balanced diet. If you eat a lot of processed foods, or are a vegan, you may be lacking in certain B vitamins, in which case adding a B-vitamin supplement to your diet can have an excellent effect on your overall health and mood.

11

Calm down with calcium

Calcium is not only essential for strong teeth and bones, it also has a soothing, calming effect and is important in maintaining a balanced mood. It is best consumed alongside vitamin D, which also helps enhance mood. Calcium is found in dairy foods such as milk, as well as in green leafy vegetables like kale and broccoli, lentils, beans, Brazil nuts and a wide variety of other vegetables. Fortified breakfast cereals and soya alternatives to dairy also provide a good source of calcium, and it is even found in tap water, especially in hard-water areas.

12

Stay hydrated

As well as being essential for good health, staying hydrated is good for your self-esteem as it helps your skin and hair look their best, which helps boost body confidence. Water also helps flush your system, keeping your bowels in working order and reducing feelings of bloating or puffiness. Drinking two litres of water each day is generally recommended for optimum health.

Cut the caffeine habit

Caffeine and other similar stimulants should be avoided as much as possible. Many of us rely on that first cup of coffee in the morning to wake us up, or a cup of tea to keep us going, but these caffeinated drinks, along with cola and foods containing caffeine, such as chocolate, could be having an adverse effect on your mood – perhaps the opposite effect to the one you intend – leaving you feeling nervous and on edge.

Drinking a caffeinated drink makes us feel more alert because it induces the initial stages of the stress reaction, boosting cortisol production. Consuming large quantities of caffeine, however, can cause the exhaustion phase of stress, and lead to anxiety. Added to this, caffeine can be very addictive, and stopping consumption of it suddenly could cause withdrawal symptoms. Try cutting down slowly to no more than 300 mg of caffeine a day, that's the equivalent of, on average, three mugs of coffee or four mugs of tea. Have fun experimenting with the huge variety of herbal teas and decaffeinated teas and coffees available in the shops.

14

Avoid alcohol

When feeling low, for example after a hard day at work, or when feeling awkward in a social situation, many people will reach for a drink to help them relax. Alcohol does have an instantly calming effect, but this is negated by its depressant qualities, and the feeling of anxiety that can be left behind once the effects wear off. Alcohol can also disturb your sleep, contrary to the popular idea of a 'nightcap'. Try to cut down your alcohol intake as much as possible, and if you do decide to have a drink, opt for a small glass of red wine, particularly Chianti, Merlot or Cabernet Sauvignon, as the beneficial plant chemicals, procyanidins, which are abundant in these wines are excellent for health, especially cardiovascular health. These wines are also rich in melatonin, the sleep hormone, and a well-rested person is more likely to feel good.

SECTION THREE:

BODY-BOOSTING EXERCISE

Feeling good about your physical abilities and your body can have an excellent effect on your self-esteem. Try these simple forms of exercise for a boost to your fitness and mood. Not only will the exercise itself produce endorphins, making you feel good inside, but seeing your body shape start to improve is bound to give your self-esteem a lift.

15

As simple as a walk

Starting to exercise can be daunting, especially if you already suffer from low self-esteem. Joining a gym or going to a group class can seem like the last thing you would want to do. However, exercise can be as simple as going for a walk. Just a half-hour walk each day can significantly improve your health and emotional well-being. You can fit this in on the way to work, at lunchtime, or whenever feels right for you. Try going for walks in daylight, in natural surroundings. The sunlight will warm your skin, and should make you feel better as it produces mood-boosting vitamin D.

Swim for self-esteem

Swimming is one of the best forms of exercise, because it not only gives you a full-body workout, but also gives you time and space to relax and unwind. As with walking, swimming is generally something you do on your own, so it's a great place to start if you are unsure about using a gym or taking part in group activities.

The rhythmic lap of the water with each stroke, and the focus on your technique and breathing, can really help to move your mind away from your concerns, giving you some quality time with yourself. This alone time can give you a chance to reflect on the positive changes you are making. Add to that the fact that floating in water is a wonderfully relaxing experience, and all part and parcel of a trip to the pool, and you've got a perfect recipe for a relaxing self-esteem boost.

17

Give yoga a chance

Whilst to some people the word 'yoga' suggests extra-bendy individuals contorting themselves gracefully into poses, the fact is this gentle, ancient form of exercise is suitable for everyone, and is a perfect self-esteem booster. Many types of exercise are competitive and can leave you feeling left behind, making you doubt your abilities, but yoga classes allow you to move at your own pace, in a way that feels right for you. Developing your strength and flexibility is likely to have a positive effect on your self-esteem, and yoga has the added benefit of allowing you to switch off from everyday thoughts and immerse yourself in the movements. Why not try a local class? Or if you don't feel ready for a group environment, there are plenty of excellent books and DVDs available, or you could look up tutorials online.

Try Pilates

Pilates is, in some ways, similar to yoga. Its gentle movements, and the focus on doing what is best for you, are certainly similar, but where yoga is about the mind-body connection, Pilates is only about the physical side of things. Pilates focuses on improving back and core strength, and on the body's alignment, leaving you walking taller and feeling more comfortable in your body. Try going along to a group class or one-to-one session with a Pilates instructor and see the benefits. Alternatively, there are many books, DVDs and online tutorials available, so you can try it out at home before committing to a class.

19

Green exercise for a natural boost

'Green exercise' is any physical activity you take part in outside, in natural surroundings. Enjoy what the great outdoors has to offer by spending more time in your garden, local park or woods. Being in natural surroundings can bring a real sense of tranquillity. Exercising outdoors, be it on the coast, through fields, or even just your own garden, can improve your mood, ease muscle tension and lower blood pressure. Feeling close to nature may give you the boost you need to keep calm under pressure, and feel balanced and content.

SECTION FOUR:

LOOK GOOD,
FEEL GREAT

It can be difficult to feel positive about yourself if you are not happy with what you see in the mirror each day. Treating yourself well and feeling comfortable about your appearance can help you feel more relaxed and self-assured, giving you an emotional boost as well as a physical one.

Clear out your wardrobe

Wearing clothes that don't fit well, or you feel uncomfortable in, can make you want to fade into the background, so try getting rid of the oldest clothes, or the ones that you feel just don't suit you any more. De-cluttering has a calming effect which can help stress levels and leave your emotions more balanced.

Make sure that the clothes you keep are the ones you really feel good in, and which make the most of your body shape. Your old ones don't have to go to landfill either; try selling them on sites like eBay, or taking them to your local charity shop where you will have the extra self-esteem boost of knowing your unwanted items have helped a charitable cause.

New for old

Once you've had your clear-out, and have your basic wardrobe down to the things you really feel good in, it's time to replace the old with something fresh. Revamping your wardrobe has multiple benefits for your self-esteem; you will most likely feel better about the way you look, and you'll be able to make the best of your body shape, whatever that may be. Choose new clothes which reflect your personality as well as being suitable for your lifestyle and career.

Remember, new to you doesn't have to mean brand new. Setting yourself up with a wardrobe to be proud of can be done on a shoestring and can be great fun. Try hunting for bargains at your local charity shops, car boot sales, and on websites such as eBay and Bigwardrobe.com.

22

Colour me happy

As well as choosing the right styles and cuts, your new wardrobe should be full of colours which suit your skin tone and boost your mood. Yellow is said to make you feel happier, blue is meant to calm and red is a power colour. If you are a fan of monochrome, you can still add these extra colours with accessories, such as a brightly coloured scarf, or with make-up, if you wear it.

A healthy glow, inside and out

Glowing, healthy skin is the basis for feeling good about the way you look. Looking in the mirror and seeing someone with a healthy appearance can have a very positive effect on your self-esteem. Put simply, when you look good, it is more likely you will feel good. To keep your skin in the best shape, make sure you cleanse and moisturise regularly. You don't need to buy expensive products as cheaper brands contain the same ingredients. Just ensure that the product is designed for your skin type, e.g. dry, oily, combination or normal.

Another important factor to remember is sunscreen. Whilst it is easy to remember to bring out the suncream on a hot day, the truth is that it should be worn most of the time, as the harmful UVA and UVB rays from the sun are still present on a cold day. In fact, you can easily become sunburnt on a snowy day, as the snow reflects the sun. The easiest way to protect your skin is to use a daytime moisturiser with added SPF.

24

Relax in the bath

A soak in the bath does wonders. As well as keeping you clean and fresh, a warm bath with your favourite bubbles or oils helps relax tense muscles and prepare the body for sleep. Being rested helps boost self-esteem. Make the most of your time in the bath; invest in some products which make you feel good, light some candles, maybe take a book with you to read whilst you soak. Take the time to really let yourself relax in the water, and use your favourite body wash to cleanse away the day. This treat will make you feel more in tune, and help you feel better both physically and emotionally.

SECTION FIVE:

DE-STRESS TO LOVE LIFE

Stress is one of the major causes of illness in the UK, and has a huge impact on self-esteem. High stress levels can leave us feeling unable to cope, which can stop us feeling good about ourselves. These stress-busting tips can help alleviate these negative feelings and leave you feeling calm, centred and self-assured.

25

Know your triggers

As individuals, we all have different needs. This also means that we have different stress factors in our lives. While there are several broad factors which can cause stress in anybody, we know ourselves best and can work out which areas affect us the most. It may be that driving to work makes you stressed, or calling your bank. Why not try cycling to work, or talking to someone in person at the bank's local branch instead? Identifying these simple triggers and making small changes is the first step to de-stressing.

Stay on budget

Financial worries are one of today's biggest stressors, with more and more people in debt and/or out of work. Taking control of your finances is excellent for your self-esteem as it helps reduce the stress that can bring your mood down, and it shows that you can take on a difficult situation and improve it.

Some simple ways to cut back on non-essential spending are: cancel any direct debits for services you do not want or need, for example, do you have a film club membership or subscriptions you hardly use? Next, look at debt; make sure you are paying off the debts with the highest interest rates first, so as to save money on interest. Getting expert advice on your debts and how to manage them is a good idea, especially if you are not sure where to start. The free Money Advice Service (www.moneyadviceservice.org.uk) can help, so this needn't be a further expense.

Finally, make sure you spend your money on the things that are most important to you, for example, is your weekly night out with friends high on your list? If so make sure you put some money aside for it. Is your car important to you? If not, you could cut the cost of running it by using public transport to get around.

27

De-stress your working day

For many people, work is the place where they experience the most stress. To make your workplace a place of calm, try adding some plants to your desk area, as they not only brighten up the place and give you some of the calming benefits of nature but also help oxygenate the environment. Further, make sure you take regular breaks from your work to avoid feeling overburdened, even if you just go to make a drink. Finally, avoid letting other people's stress rub off on you. Stress can be 'caught' from your colleagues, so if a workmate is complaining and being overly negative, either move the conversation away from the subject, or if you can't, excuse yourself and spend some time away from them. Though it's not possible to remove all stressors from your working day, reducing them in this way will help you feel more in control and confident in your ability to face new challenges.

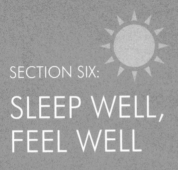

SECTION SIX:

SLEEP WELL, FEEL WELL

A lack of sleep can leave us feeling unmotivated and sluggish, and many aspects of our lives can fall by the wayside. Being well rested makes us feel calmer and more self-assured; try these tips to improve your bedtime routine and see what good comes of it.

28

Know what's normal for you

Though the average adult needs eight hours' sleep each night, we are not all average. Some need more and some need less. Knowing what is normal for you can help you be sure that you are not oversleeping or getting too little sleep, either of which can be a source of stress and concern. It may help to keep a sleep diary, or to use an app which tells you the optimum time to wake up taking into consideration your chosen bedtime. Many apps give several options based on the number of full sleep cycles you require.

Avoid screens

We spend a large amount of time in front of screens each day – computers, tablets, televisions and smartphones are core parts of most people's lives. These sorts of backlit screens, however, are detrimental to our sleep cycles. It may seem like watching a film or reading an article on your tablet are good ways to unwind before bed, but these activities make the brain more active, and therefore make it harder to switch off at night. Bright screens halt the production of the sleep hormone, melatonin, by making our brains think it is daytime and time to be awake. Instead, try reading a book in gentle light, or listening to some calming music, to help you drift off.

Make your bedroom the best room

Poor-quality sleep can have as much of an effect on self-esteem as lack of sleep. To help ensure that you feel great, and ready to start the day each morning, make your bedroom into a sanctuary where you can escape the worries of the day. Experts advise that bedrooms should be for sleep and sex only, so remove all distractions – do away with the computers and televisions, and even, if you can, your mobile phone. Keep paperwork out of the bedroom by opening your post elsewhere, and save important discussions for other rooms. Finally, make sure your space is tidy and inviting, and soon you will be sleeping soundly and your self-esteem will be thanking you for it.

31

If in doubt, count sheep!

The idea of visualisation may sound 'New Age' to some, but people have been using it for many years. The old advice of 'count sheep until you fall asleep' is a form of visualisation – you see the sheep jumping over the fence one by one and count them, feeling sleepier as the numbers get higher.

Other visualisations may help. Rather than visualising energetic sheep bouncing over a fence, for example, why not visualise sleeping sheep? See yourself floating over a night-time meadow, passing dozing sheep one at a time. The more sheep you see, the more you want to lie down in the soft grass and rest. These sleeping sheep may help you get to sleep better than their wide-awake counterparts. Of course, this sort of visualisation can use any symbol, perhaps something you find particularly relaxing; sheep are just a starting point.

Find ways to make your night quieter

Night-time noise can be a big cause of sleep disturbance. This can be anything from a ticking clock, to sirens outside, to a snoring partner. It is likely you will already know which noises usually wake you up. In an ideal world, you would remove these sounds completely, but, of course, this is not always possible. There are many things you can easily do, however, like removing the battery from a ticking clock at night, or fixing that dripping tap, which can help improve the quality of your sleep and, with it, help you feel more equipped for the challenges of the day ahead.

Keep it dark

Like sound, light can cause disturbed sleep and early waking, which often leads to poor-quality rest and irritability, leaving you feeling ill-prepared for the day ahead. While darkness causes your brain to produce melatonin, the hormone that makes you feel sleepy, light helps it produce serotonin, too much of which will make you feel more awake.

To help keep your bedroom as dark as possible, make sure any electrical items such as stereos are turned off, not on standby, as the lights from their displays may keep you awake. You should also choose thick, dark curtains or blinds, to ensure outside light does not intrude and wake you. If light is a particular nuisance for you, try using blackout curtains or blinds.

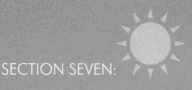

SECTION SEVEN:

GOAL-SETTING FOR GREATNESS

Knowing you want to achieve more is a positive thing, but it can become a stressor if you are not sure how you are going to achieve your goals, or even what it is you want. Setting goals and working towards them brings a sense of achievement, which is sure to boost self-esteem.

Start with a to-do list

It can often seem like there is too much to do, with not enough hours in the day, which makes thinking about setting and achieving goals seem like an impossible task. Sometimes there really may be too much to do in one day, but getting organised will help you feel confident in your ability to prioritise tasks and complete them on time, which is sure to boost your self-esteem. Simple as it may sound, if you are unsure about your organisational skills, then a simple to-do list may well be the best thing to try. A notepad or a piece of paper will do the trick, or you could invest in an attractive book to write your lists in. They can be as simple or as detailed as you like, the main thing is that they work well for you, and that you enjoy ticking off each task as you complete it.

35

Make your goals personal

Goal-setting is key to success and therefore to building up your self-esteem. It may be that you want to set small goals to help break down bigger tasks, or it may be that you have long-term aims that you want to make reality. The most important thing, no matter how big or small the goal, is that it is personal to you; your needs, lifestyle and interests. If you choose to do something because you feel you 'should', or because it is what others want you to do, the chances are you will not have the motivation to make it all the way. Instead, try to make sure your aims reflect what you really love – be it food, family, art or nature – and see how easily you work towards these goals that focus on your own happiness.

36

Be SMART

While setting challenging goals is an important part of achieving what we want in life, many of us set unrealistic goals. Self-esteem can take a hit if it seems like your aspirations are impossible to reach, as you are not managing your goals. One positive way to ensure that your aims will work for you is by making them SMART (specific, measurable, attainable, relevant and time-bound). This means you should know exactly what it is you want to achieve (S), you should be able to measure your progress (M), it should be possible for you to achieve it, though not too easy (A), it should relate to your wider aims (R), and you should know when you want to have reached your goal by (T). Why not try setting yourself some SMART goals in the notes pages at the end of this book?

There's no such thing as failure

It is quite possible that, even if you set the most relevant, realistic goals, you may not achieve them in the way or the time you wanted to. Life may throw something unexpected in your path, which stops you from achieving what you want, when you want. This is not failure. Feeling like you have failed is bound to lead to low mood, and can often come about if things haven't quite gone according to plan. However, the best thing to do is to draw a mental line under it, learn from what has happened and try again. As long as you are still trying, you are working towards your long-term aims, and as long as you are doing that, you are never truly failing.

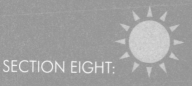

SECTION EIGHT:

THE BRAIN IS A POWERFUL THING

Your thoughts have a strong influence on the way you feel and behave. The tips in this section show you ways to understand and challenge your thoughts, and build a more positive self-image to help improve your self-esteem.

Understand what a thought is

Every person has as many as 50,000 thoughts every day. These can be simple things like 'I wonder if my train will be on time', or they can be powerful, such as 'I'm not skilled enough for my job'. Part of the concept of mindfulness, a powerful technique developed from Buddhist teachings, is recognising thoughts and seeing that they do not need to control the way you feel and behave. Repeating the same negative thought pattern for many years may have had a detrimental effect on your self-esteem, but once you can recognise this negativity as simply a thought, with no substance, you can begin to challenge it and rebuild your self-belief.

No comparison

Many people compare themselves with others and conclude that they are imperfect, rather than focusing on their own qualities and recognising the positives. Comparing yourself with others is not a good idea, as our opinions of others are unlikely to match their opinions of themselves. The person you think is better at their job than you may in fact be insecure about their abilities, and the person you think is more attractive than you may spend hours every day getting ready before showing their face in public. Try instead focusing on yourself; there may be some aspects of your life you want to improve, but only do so because it will make you happier, not because you want to be like someone else.

40

Ask yourself 'why?'

One of the key ways to challenge the negative thoughts about yourself which can impact on your self-esteem is to ask 'why?' For example, the commonly held negative thought 'I'm not good enough' can make you worried about many aspects of your life – perhaps you feel you are not good enough at your job, not a good enough friend, not a good enough homemaker. Now is the time to ask yourself why you feel this way – can you find five genuine reasons why you are not good enough? It is likely you will struggle to find any real reasons. Let logic prevail: if the only way you can answer this simple question is with 'because I know it's true' or by stating that minor incidents from the past make it so, you can see that really, the assumption that you are not good enough is just a thought that has become ingrained, and which can be removed, allowing you to build a more positive self-image.

41

Would someone else say that to you?

Coming to terms with tip 40 can be particularly hard if your self-esteem is at an all-time low, because you may strongly believe the thoughts you are trying to remove from your life. You may even find reasons, however spurious, that such thoughts are 'true'. If this is the case, try this simple exercise: think about your best friend, sibling or colleague; somebody you respect. Now, do you think this person would agree with your negative thoughts? Would they say the sort of things to you that you are saying to yourself? And finally, would you tell the other person what you are telling yourself? The likelihood is that your answer is no. You may even be shocked at the thought; why would you treat someone that way? And why would someone be cruel to you? The answer is, you are being cruel to yourself. The lesson here is to treat yourself like your best friend. Allow yourself the same consideration you would want from and give to another person, and be kind to yourself.

42

Speak with confidence

When lacking self-esteem, it is possible to come across as being unsure of yourself, especially in the way you speak. Public speaking, in particular, can be very difficult, and worry may cause your voice to become higher pitched as your vocal cords tighten. You may also end up speaking more quietly, less evenly and in a way which lacks authority. This can cause a vicious cycle of low self-esteem, as you may not feel listened to or respected. To remedy this, try practising a more powerful voice; let your tone be deeper, and your words be slow and steady. Say what you want to say, like you mean it, and see the difference it can make. If you try this in front of a mirror it can be even more helpful, as you get used to seeing yourself talk, and act as your own audience. Seeing yourself progress to speaking calmly and with authority can help overcome nerves if you have to speak publicly.

Tell yourself you can

Positive self-talk is key to breaking a cycle of negative thoughts, so why not try using mantras to break the cycle? A mantra is a positive phrase that you repeat to yourself, confirming your positive thoughts. Mantras can be thought, or said out loud; many people believe that actually saying your mantra out loud makes it more effective, as vocalising something gives it more substance. You can also write your chosen mantra down and put it somewhere you are likely to see it, such as the kitchen or bathroom. Regularly repeating your chosen mantra can help you reaffirm your faith in yourself and your abilities.

Focus on your abilities

Everybody has their own personal set of skills and abilities. When your self-esteem is low, it can be hard to focus on these and you can start to feel like you aren't good at much at all. When this happens, try the simple exercise of writing down all the things you're good at. This doesn't have to be anything huge, you could start with something like 'I bake great cakes' and go from there. If you find this very hard, try asking a friend or trusted colleague what they think your abilities are. You could use the notes pages at the end of this book to write them down, so that you can look back at them if you are feeling low, having a bad day or doubting yourself; they might help to inject some positivity into your day.

CONSIDER COMPLEMENTARY THERAPIES

Complementary therapies are widely available and can be an excellent way to boost your mood and strengthen your self-esteem, whilst giving you some 'me time' and helping you to relax.

45

Aromatherapy mood boost

Aromatherapy is an age-old therapy which uses essential oils to help calm or stimulate the mind and body. To enhance your mood, try using stimulating oils such as geranium, rosemary or peppermint, or uplifting scents such as rose, bergamot or neroli. These can be used traditionally for massage, steam inhalation or as bath oils, but they can also be used around your home or workplace to help bring you back to yourself throughout the day. Try sprinkling some drops on a pomander to hang in your wardrobe, or using your favourite oil on some unscented potpourri.

46

Reflexology for balance and calm

Reflexology is similar to acupressure, using stimulation of certain points to help the flow of energy through the body. These points are found on the feet, hands and face, but practitioners will usually use the feet as these are more sensitive, and are believed to have points which relate to every part of the body. Stimulating these points is meant to release energy blockages in the related body part, therefore facilitating the free flow of energy through that body part, and helping to reduce illness. The relaxation alone can help reduce stress and make you feel more balanced. For practicality, if you decide to try this on yourself, it may be easier to use your hands, and, although reflexology can be self-practiced, it is more beneficial to visit a trained reflexologist for treatment. Look up your local natural health centre for more information.

47

Try EFT

Emotional freedom techniques (EFT) are a set of techniques that use tapping to unlock blocked energy, therefore promoting the improvement of health and well-being. Like acupuncture and acupressure, the techniques are based on the idea of 'qi' or energy moving through 'meridians' in the body. The concept is that blockages in these meridians can cause illness and emotional problems. With EFT, you hold on to the negative emotion or thought which is blocking the flow of energy through your body, whilst tapping on the relevant body point, then you do the same again, only this time using a positive statement to replace the negative thought. This therapy is supposed to be particularly good for self-esteem issues and can be used alongside the mindfulness tips outlined in earlier chapters. EFT can easily be tried at home, with online tutorials and illustrations readily available.

48

Massage away the tension

A good massage will leave you feeling relaxed and ready to face new challenges. As well as promoting healthy blood flow and relaxing the muscles, being massaged gives you time to just focus on you. Look up a local massage therapist, or ask a friend or partner to give your shoulders, back or feet a calming, soothing rub. Alternatively, you can try self-massage on your hands, feet, legs or scalp.

Using aromatherapy oils such as lavender or neroli will help to make this experience even more calming, and will help boost your mood.

49

Supplementary help

As an extra way to balance your mood and improve feelings of self-esteem, supplements can be very helpful. If you talk to someone at your local health food shop or natural pharmacy, they will be able to point you in the right direction. Some of the most effective herbal supplements for self-esteem are those which calm the mind and ease feelings of anxiety and stress; two remedies which are very popular are passiflora (passion flower) and valerian. These are widely available and can be taken as a tincture or a tablet, or drunk as an infusion. As a milder remedy, try chamomile tea, which is renowned for its ability to relax and soothe.

50

And finally…
seeing your doctor

If you feel your self-esteem has reached an all-time low, and/or it is having a negative effect on your life, it is worth speaking to your doctor. Although complementary therapies can help a great deal, sometimes a medical opinion is required, as low self-esteem can be a sign of more serious issues. It may be that your doctor recommends a talking therapy such as cognitive behavioural therapy (CBT), or medication, to help you feel better until your situation improves. Remember, the doctor is there to help you, so tell them everything and hopefully you will be feeling the benefit before long.

Notes

50 TIPS
TO HELP YOU
DE-STRESS

Anna Barnes

50 TIPS TO HELP YOU DE-STRESS

Anna Barnes

ISBN: 978-1-84953-402-4

Hardback

£5.99

No matter how hard we try, there are times for all of us when the stresses and strains of daily life start to pile up. This book of simple, easy-to-follow tips gives you the tools and techniques you need to recognise your stress triggers and learn to take life as it comes, with a calm and balanced outlook.

50 TIPS
TO HELP YOU
SLEEP WELL

Anna Barnes

50 TIPS TO HELP YOU SLEEP WELL

Anna Barnes

ISBN: 978-1-84953-401-7

Hardback

£5.99

There are times for all of us when, no matter how many sheep we have counted, falling asleep just isn't as easy as it should be. This book of simple, easy-to-follow tips provides you with the tools and techniques needed to understand your sleep patterns, and to make changes that will steer you on the path towards restful sleep.

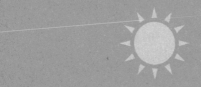

If you're interested in finding out more about our books,
find us on Facebook at **Summersdale Publishers**
and follow us on Twitter at **@Summersdale**.

www.summersdale.com